Hot and Bothered At 3am

How To Stop Menopausal Night Sweats In 7 Days Or Less

By Angela Knight

I0435936

Table Of Contents

Introduction 4

   Hormones - The Number 1 Cause Of Night Sweats 4

   Common Symptoms Of Night Sweats 7

   10 Contributory Factors 10

   Night Sweats Before Menopause? It Can Happen! 13

The Top 3 Strategies For Stopping Night Sweats 15

   1. Lifestyle Changes 16

   2. Alternative Medicine....................................17

   3. Drugs And Surgery 19

10 Easy Lifestyle Changes You Can Make To Stop Night
Sweats 20

   1. Exercise...20

   2. Weight Loss 21

   3. Diet..22

   4. Deep Breathing 23

   5. Stay Comfortable 24

   6. Dietary Supplements 25

   7. Phytoestrogens 26

   8. Acupuncture 27

   9. Homeopathy 28

   10. Yoga 29

12 Secret Remedies For Night Sweats 30

1. Black Cohosh...30

2. Vitamin E..31

3. Flaxseed...31

4. Pycnogenol...32

5. Minerals..33

6. Soy...34

7. Sage...35

8. Berries..36

9. Teas And Tinctures...37

10. Licorice...37

11. Macafem Route...37

12. Dong Quai...38

The 10 Most Effective Drugs And Surgical Treatments For
Excessive Sweating...39

1. Hormone Replacement Therapy......................................39

2. Antidepressants...41

3. Gabapentin...42

4. Clonidine..42

5. Megestrol Acetate (Megace)...42

6. Botox...43

7. Sweat Gland Surgery..43

8. Endoscopic Thoracic Sympathectomy.............................43

9. Lumbar Sympathectomy...44

10. Local Anesthetics...44

Introduction

Hormones - The Number 1 Cause Of Night Sweats

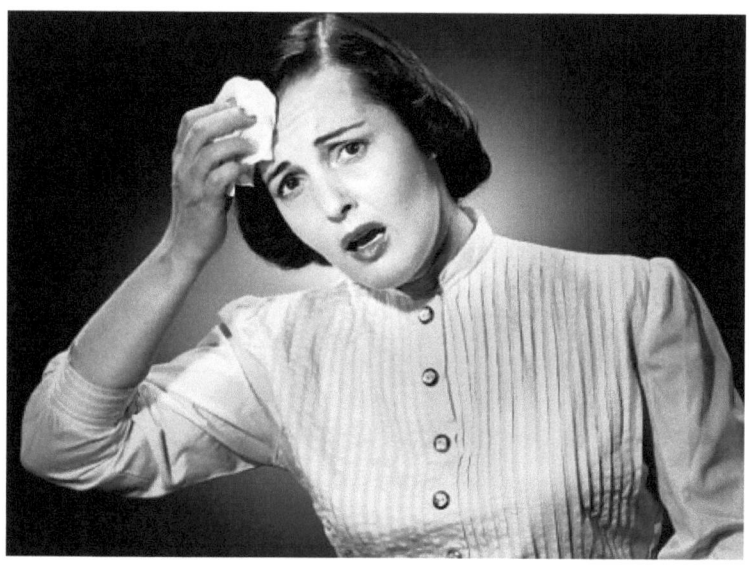

In addition to hot flashes, many menopausal women experience the symptom's nocturnal accomplice known as night sweats. You wake up in the middle of the night cold and clammy, your heart pounding, and the sheets drenched in sweat. It's hard to calm down and get comfortable again, and it's impossible not to be irritated by the interruption to a good night's sleep. So why do women in menopause have night sweats, and, more importantly, is there anything that can be done about them?

Hot flashes and night sweats are caused by a complex interaction that involves fluctuating estrogen levels;

the hypothalamus (a region of the brain that regulates body temperature); norepinephrine, a key brain chemical, and specialized receptors in the brain; and the body's blood vessels and sweat glands.

During menopause, estrogen levels fluctuate. The hypothalamus can become confused by these changes in estrogen levels. Like a faulty thermostat, the hypothalamus may respond to the changes in estrogen as if it senses an increase in your body's temperature. In an attempt to cool you down, the hypothalamus sets off a cascade of events, including dilating blood vessels to release heat (which you feel as a hot flash) and triggering sweat glands (which you feel as sudden, intense perspiration). The result is you wake up drenched and chilly, with a speeding heart and a sensation of anxiety.

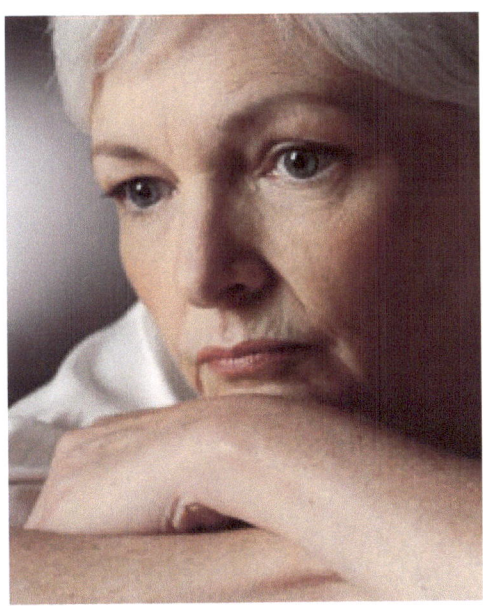

While night sweats can be uncomfortable and disruptive, they don't usually signal a more serious underlying condition. In fact, night sweats are one of the most common symptoms of menopause, which typically begins in a woman's late 40s to early 50s. Scientific studies suggest that as many as 75% of menopausal women experience night sweats. When a woman approaches menopause, she may have many questions about the potential symptoms, including night sweats. Understanding what to expect, why these symptoms occur, and how to manage them can help a woman best prepare for this transitional period.

Common Symptoms Of Night Sweats

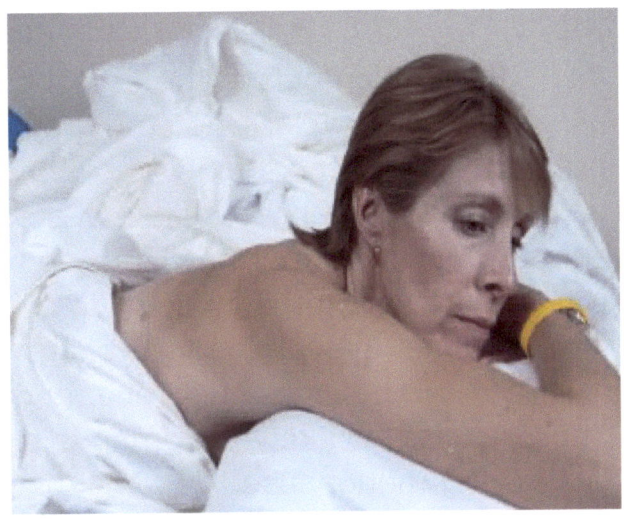

Signs and symptoms of night sweats often resemble those of daytime hot flashes, but are chiefly characterized by excessive sweating. The intensity of night sweats symptoms typically varies depending on the woman. For example, while a majority of menopausal women will experience night sweats, only one in four will experience them severely. Sudden intense heat, perspiration, heart palpitations, nausea, headaches, flushing, chills, wet clothing/bedding, interrupted sleep are all common symptoms.

The symptoms of night sweats can drastically disturb sleep patterns, making it difficult to get a good night's rest. Because of this, women who suffer from night sweats often experience insomnia, sleep disorders, trouble concentrating, exhaustion, irritability and heightened levels of stress.

Many women in their 40s and 50s develop night sweats, which often begin before the actual cessation of a woman's menstrual cycle. One study found that approximately 19% of women aged 40 to 55 who still had regular periods experienced night sweats. Most women begin to develop symptoms three to ten years before actual menopause, during the span of time called perimenopause. Research shows that not all women are affected the same. Age, race, and other factors can influence how likely a woman is to develop night sweats during menopause.

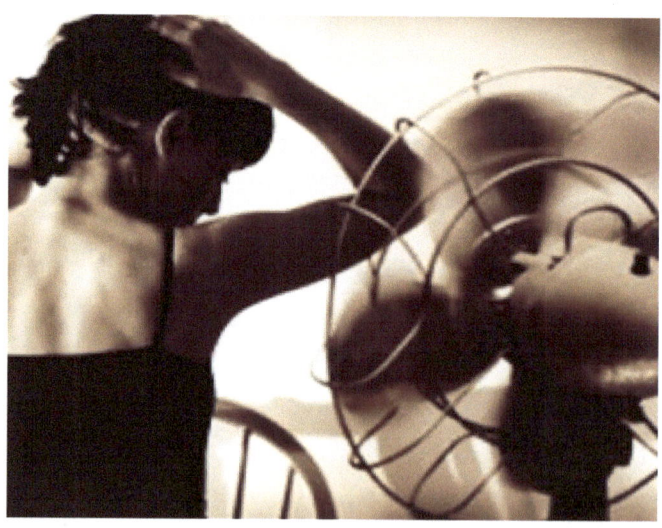

One study found that younger women are significantly more likely than older women to experience night sweats. Another found that only 10% of patients older than 64 had night sweats. Studies have found that the prevalence of night sweats varies by race. One study found that 3 in 4 Caucasian women experience night sweats. Another found that African-American women were more likely to have night sweats than Caucasian or Hispanic women. Asian women were least likely to report night sweats.

10 Contributory Factors

While the most common cause of night sweats during the menopausal transition is a fluctuation in hormone levels, night sweats can also be a symptom of other medical conditions. To determine what is causing night sweats in a particular individual, a doctor must obtain a detailed medical history and order tests to decide if an underlying medical condition is responsible. Some of the known conditions that can cause night sweats are:

1. Menopause- The hot flushes that accompany the menopausal transition can occur at night and cause sweating. This is a very common cause of night sweats in perimenopausal women.

2. Idiopathic hyperhidrosis - Idiopathic hyperhidrosis is a condition in which the body chronically produces too much sweat without any identifiable medical cause.

3. Infections - Classically, tuberculosis is the infection most commonly associated with night sweats. In 2002, TB affected more than 15,000 people in the United States. It can be fatal when untreated. Among its symptoms are a fever, a cough, and of course night sweats. However, bacterial infections, such as endocarditis (inflammation of the heart valves), osteomyelitis (inflammation within the bones), and abscesses all may result in night sweats.

Night sweats are also a symptom of AIDS virus (HIV) infection.

4. Cancers - Night sweats are an early symptom of some cancers. The most common type of cancer associated with night sweats is lymphoma. However, people who have an undiagnosed cancer frequently have other symptoms as well, such as unexplained weight loss and fevers.

5. Medications - Taking certain medication can lead to night sweats. In cases without other physical symptoms or signs of tumour or infection, medication is often determined to be the cause of night sweats. Antidepressant medication is a common type of medication that can lead to night sweats. Medicines taken to lower fever such as aspirin and paracetamol can sometimes lead to sweating. Other types of drugs can cause flushing, which, as mentioned above, may be confused with night sweats. Some of the many drugs that can cause flushing include:

Niacin (taken in the higher doses used for lipid disorders), Tamoxifen, Hydralazine, Nitroglycerine, and Sildenafil (Viagra). Many other drugs not mentioned above, including cortisone medications such as prednisone and prednisolone, may also be associated with flushing or night sweats.

6. Hypoglycaemia- Sometimes low blood glucose can cause sweating. People who are taking insulin or oral diabetes medications may experience hypoglycaemia at night that is accompanied by sweating.

7. Hormone disorders - Sweating or flushing can be seen with several hormone disorders, including pheochromocytoma, carcinoid syndrome, and hyperthyroidism.

8. Neurological conditions - Uncommonly, neurological conditions including autonomic dysreflexia, post-traumatic syringomyelia, stroke, and autonomic neuropathy may cause increased sweating and possibly lead to night sweats.

9. Fevers - There can be many reasons for a fever. But as your body temperature begins break, you often sweat profusely, which is your body's way of getting rid of the excess heat. This is normal; however repeated episodes of fever then sweating and chills can mean a serious infection or other illness.

10. Withdrawals - When people quit taking certain drugs or alcohol, their body goes through withdrawals. Along with sweating, symptoms of withdrawal include shaking, anxiety, nausea, fever and hallucinations.

Night Sweats Before Menopause? It Can Happen!

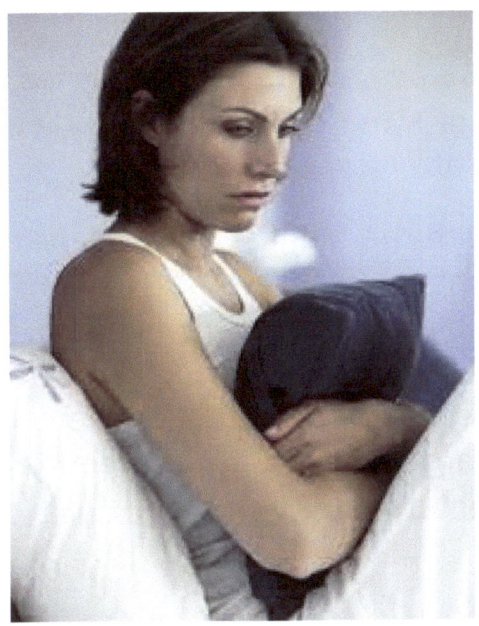

A new study has revealed that more than half of middle-aged women who still have regular cycles have hot flashes. According to a survey of some 1,500 women, Asian and Hispanic women are less likely to have them than white women, but compared with previous studies, the figures are surprisingly high.

The survey, conducted by researchers at Group Health (a large healthcare system in the Pacific Northwest) and Fred Hutchinson Cancer Research Center in Seattle, Washington, consisted of a diverse group of women, including whites, blacks, Hawaiian/Pacific Islanders, women of mixed ethnicity, Vietnamese, Filipinos, Japanese, East Indians, Chinese, and other

Asians. The women were 45 to 56 years old, had regular cycles, had not skipped periods, and were not taking hormones.

A surprising 55 percent of them reported having hot flashes or night sweats. (Previous studies pegged the highest rates at below 50 percent.)

The groups with the highest proportions reporting hot flashes or night sweats were Native Americans (67 percent) and black (61 percent) women, but the differences between these groups and white women weren`t statistically significant. 58 percent of white women, the largest ethnic group, reported having hot flashes or night sweats.

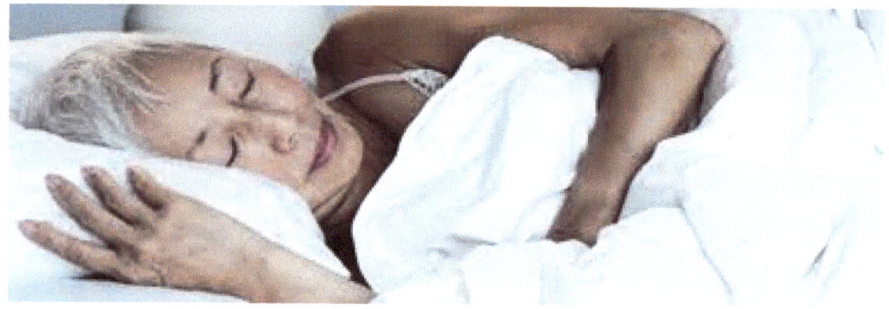

Compared with them, Asian and Hispanic women were significantly less likely to have these symptoms. Among Asian women, 31 percent of Filipino, 26 percent of Japanese, 25 percent of East Indian, 23 percent of "other Asian," and 18 percent of Chinese women reported having hot flashes or night sweats. 26 percent of Hispanic women reported these symptoms.

The Top 3 Strategies For Stopping Night Sweats

When it comes to night sweats treatment, it is important to be patient in finding the right route to relief. Because the pattern and severity of night sweats is different for everyone, each menopausal woman may need to do a bit of experimenting in order to determine what works best for her. What might work for a few weeks may not prove to be a long term solution. For some women finding relief is easy, while for others it might take a little more perseverance.

In order to determine the best night sweats treatment, it is a good idea to begin by keeping track of the circumstances around which night sweats occur. For example, making note of the time of the episode, emotional state (e.g. stress level), food and drink consumed prior to bed, clothing worn, and sleeping conditions, etc. This information can alert a woman as to what is triggering her night sweats, which may help her determine what treatment is most effective.

A woman wishing to treat night sweats has three categories, or levels, of treatment available to her: (1) Lifestyle changes, (2) Alternative medicine and (3) Drugs and surgery. These three levels of approaches are not mutually exclusive. A woman may use different approaches at different times or any combination of them, depending on the duration and severity of symptoms. Today more and more women find that dealing with menopause symptoms is best accomplished via a combination of healthy lifestyle and alternative treatments.

1. Lifestyle Changes

Lifestyle changes are the first level of treatment available to women wishing to rid themselves of night sweats. While these changes are usually cost-free and virtually risk-free, they do require the greatest amount of self-discipline. Believe it or not, daily behaviours can have a significant impact on a woman's experience of night sweats. For example, eating a spicy dinner, having one too many glasses of wine, or experiencing increased stress due to work pressure or family obligations can trigger night sweats. Lifestyle adjustments are two-pronged: they aid women in avoiding triggers and also serve to increase overall health

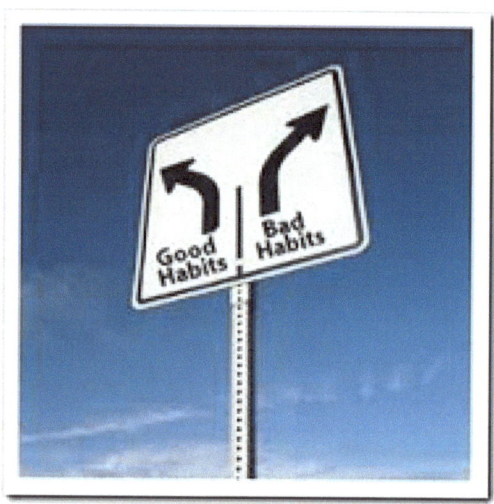

Making lifestyle changes is easier said than done. It may be possible to skip that extra glass of wine, but virtually impossible to avoid work-related stress. It can also be difficult to suddenly and drastically change habits and preferences you may have had your whole life. Moreover, while these changes will help alleviate many symptoms, they do not address the cause of night sweats: hormonal imbalance. Fortunately, alternative medicine treatments are available to treat the root hormonal imbalance. These natural treatments have a much lower risk of side effects, compared to medical hormonal treatments.

2. Alternative Medicine

This level of approach can involve several different therapies. Herbal remedies are the most popular, though in addition women may turn to such techniques as acupuncture, biofeedback, massage, homeopathy, or hypnosis. All of these can be effective options, though most women find that herbal remedies are the easiest alternative treatment to follow, as the others require a greater time and monetary commitment. In addition, herbal remedies are the only viable option to treat the hormonal imbalance directly at its source.

In the case of herbal remedies, there are two types of herbs that can be used for treating night sweats: phytoestrogenic and non-estrogenic herbs. Phytoestrogenic herbs contain estrogenic components produced by plants. These herbs, at first, treat the hormonal imbalance by introducing these plant-based estrogens into the body. However as a result of adding outside hormones, a woman's body may become less capable of producing estrogen on its own. This causes a further decrease of the body's own hormone levels.

By contrast, non-estrogenic herbs, as the name suggests, don't contain any estrogen. These herbs stimulate a woman's hormone production by nourishing the pituitary and endocrine glands, causing them to more efficiently produce natural hormones. This ultimately results in balancing not only estrogen, but also progesterone and testosterone. Non-estrogenic herbs can be considered the safest way to treat night sweats naturally as the body creates its own hormones and doesn't require any outside assistance.

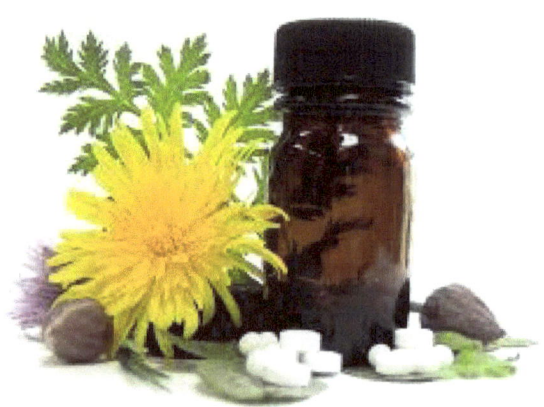

Non-estrogenic herbs help restore natural hormones in women. Unlike hormone drugs, which are basically resumed in taking synthetic hormones, they act totally different in your body. They nourish and stimulate your own natural hormone production, by inducing the optimal functioning of the pituitary and endocrine glands.

A combination of approaches is usually the most effective route to take. Lifestyle changes combined with alternative medicine will most likely be the best way to alleviate the symptoms of this hormonal imbalance. While this approach is optimal for many women, others will find that they want or need to go to the third level of treatment.

3. Drugs And Surgery

Interventions at the third level involve the highest risk and often the highest costs. For the 70 to 75 per cent of women who have menopausal hot flushes, some of whom experience several attacks a week for four or more years, there is a bewildering range of over-the-counter and prescription treatments available. Many have been found to be effective, but large numbers have not, and in some cases the placebo or dummy treatment has been shown to be as effective as the therapy on trial.

10 Easy Lifestyle Changes You Can Make To Stop Night Sweats

1. Exercise

Some research indicates that increasing cardio-respiratory fitness, including walking and yoga, could be a way to reduce menopausal symptoms. One study found, for example, that women who engaged in regular physical activity had fewer and less severe night sweats. Another study concluded that overweight women were more likely to have hot flashes than their slimmer peers. Recent developments suggest it may be more complicated than that — age is a factor, too — but experts agree that getting active is good for your health regardless.

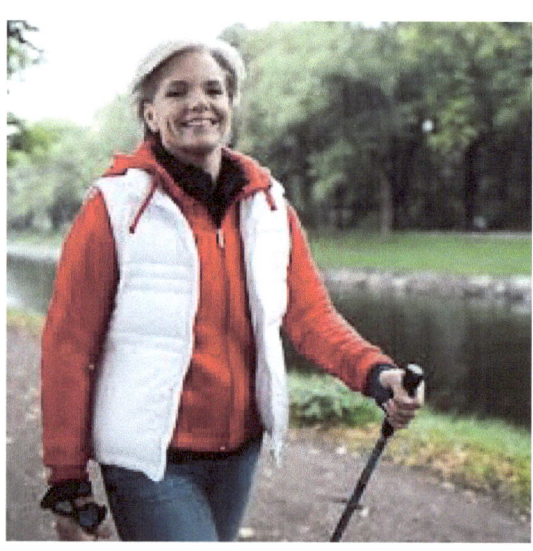

A research team from the University of Pittsburgh asked 52 women—all transitioning through menopause—to keep a sleep diary. The researchers also tracked the women's exercise habits and menopause-related symptoms. Here's what they discovered: The more women moved—whether exercising away from home, or completing physically active household chores like preparing meals or caregiving for family members—the sounder they slept, according to the study.

While these findings are promising, it's not clear exactly how physical activity might squelch hot flashes and other symptoms of menopause. There's a whole lot of research that shows physically active people tend to sleep better at night, and the study indicates this is also true for woman suffering from hot flashes.

And no, you don't have to hit the weights or elliptical machine to get some ZZZs tonight. In fact, past studies have found intense exercise increases core body temperature, and so may trigger menopausal symptoms like hot flashes. Simply staying on your feet and being active—even at home—is enough to improve your sleep.

2. Weight Loss

At the end of a 12-month study period, women who lost at least 10 pounds (or 10% of their body weight) were 23% more likely to experience fewer or no hot flashes, found a study funded by Kaiser Permanente. It may sound obvious, but fat locks in body heat. And since night flashes are, essentially, your body's attempt to cool itself off, shedding a little excess insulation can help keep you cool and reduce your menopause-related symptoms.

3. Diet

Eat more fruit. The same Kaiser Permanente study also directed women to eat more fiber-rich foods, especially fruit and whole grains. Although the researchers attributed most of the drop in hot flashes to weight loss, they said it was also possible the improved fiber intake may have helped reduce the frequency of menopause symptoms.

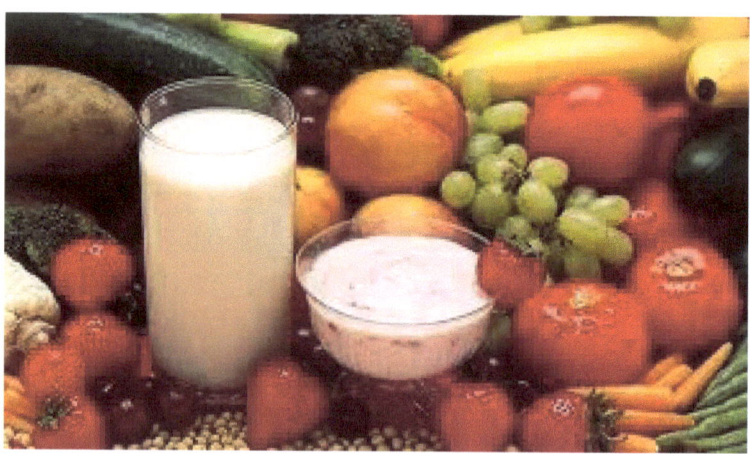

When it comes to food, you should avoid spicy foods, stews, soups and caffeinated foods; and when it comes to drinks, you should avoid caffeinated drinks, alcohol, and hot drinks. Cigarette smoke should be avoided, as well.

Caffeine is a stimulant that increases your metabolic rate. People who use caffeine experience increased alertness, blood pressure, and breathing rate. However, caffeine can also makes many people feel jittery, and sometimes unable to sleep. Long-term use can lead to insomnia, nervousness, dehydration, fatigue, and excessive sweating.

Alcohol acts as a depressant to the central nervous system. It causes sweating, and can mess with the temperature regulating mechanism in the brain.

4. Deep Breathing

Deep breathing, or relaxation breathing or paced respiration, involves breathing in deeply and exhaling at an even pace. You should slowly breathe in through your nose. With a hand on your stomach right below your ribs, you should first feel your stomach push your hand out, and then your chest should fill. Slowly exhale through your mouth, first letting your lungs empty and then feeling your stomach sink back.

Abdominal breathing exercises can halve the number of attacks. At the time of writing, a much larger clinical trial of breathing exercises is underway as researchers look for new treatments for the condition. In new research at Indiana University, doctors are recruiting around 200 women for the biggest trial yet of slow deep breathing. It follows a number of small studies which have shown that it can be highly effective. Results from a study at Wayne State

University in America, show that paced respiration reduced hot flush frequency by around 50 per cent.

Deep breathing can help greatly when it comes to stress, too. Just practice breathing deeply for fifteen minutes every morning and every night, and you are sure to keep your night sweats at bay.

5. Stay Comfortable

Simple measures, such as minimal bed clothes, keeping room temperatures down, windows open and a fan to hand, can be helpful, together with wearing natural fibres and layered clothing that can be easily removed. There are cooling scarves available using newer textile technology and also pillows called 'chillow pillows' – both can be soothing and bought online.

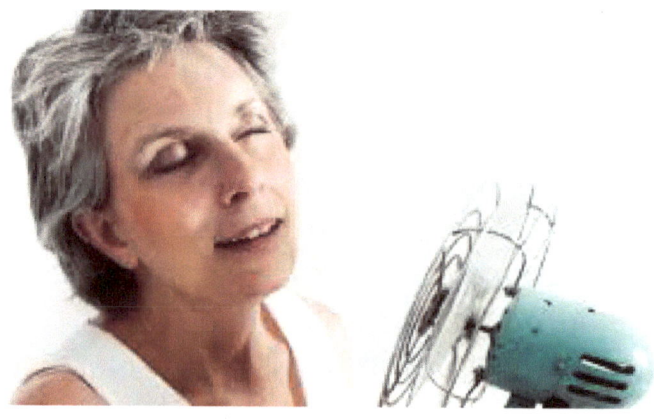

Put a fan in your bedroom to keep air cool and circulating. And consider wearing "wicking" pajamas. Made from the same material used in hiking gear, this type of pajama can draw sweat away from your skin, easing any clamminess and helping you to sleep on peacefully. Some women find that taking a tepid bath in the morning for 20 minutes prevents hot flashes all day long.

6. Dietary Supplements

Research has looked at whether dietary supplements can help flushes and sweats. Multivitamin and mineral products, which are specifically formulated for menopausal women, are widely available. Anecdotally, they can improve flushes and sweats, particularly if there is a known nutritional deficiency due to a poor diet or if there are digestive and/or absorption problems. Rather than taking supplements, however, aim for a varied diet, eating at least five portions of fruit, salad and vegetables daily and plenty of wholegrain, high-fibre foods. Also try cutting down on saturated fats, increasing mono and polyunsaturated fats instead.

Functional foods potentially have beneficial health effects and include probiotics and vitamin and mineral- enriched products. However, the only ones that may help to reduce hot flushes are products containing probiotics with phytoestrogens.

7. Phytoestrogens

Many products based on soy, red clover and other sources of phytoestrogens (plant oestrogens) are available for hot flushes. Always buy a reputable brand with a guarantee of quality. Since 2011, a number of products have registered with the Medicines and Healthcare products Regulatory Agency (MHRA) to meet the required standard relating to quality, safety and effectiveness – look for the Traditional Herbal Registration (THR) certification mark on the packaging.

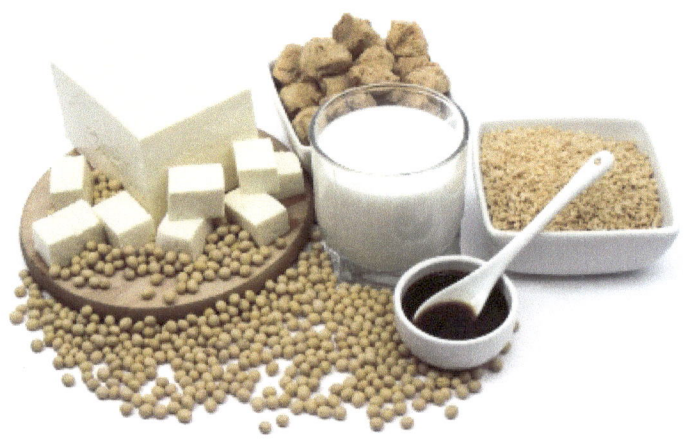

The effectiveness of phytoestrogens has varied in studies, probably because of the range of products involved. One study in 2011 showed that 80mg of isoflavones daily reduced flushes and improved sleep significantly but only after four months of use. Phytoestrogens need to be broken down in the gut to be absorbed and become active; eating probiotic live yoghurt can help this process in some women. Phytoestrogens appear to be safe in healthy women.

8. Acupuncture

A number of studies have suggested that acupuncture can reduce hot flushes and other menopause-related symptoms. For most women, acupuncture is safe, but it is important to find a qualified therapist with experience in treating menopausal symptoms.

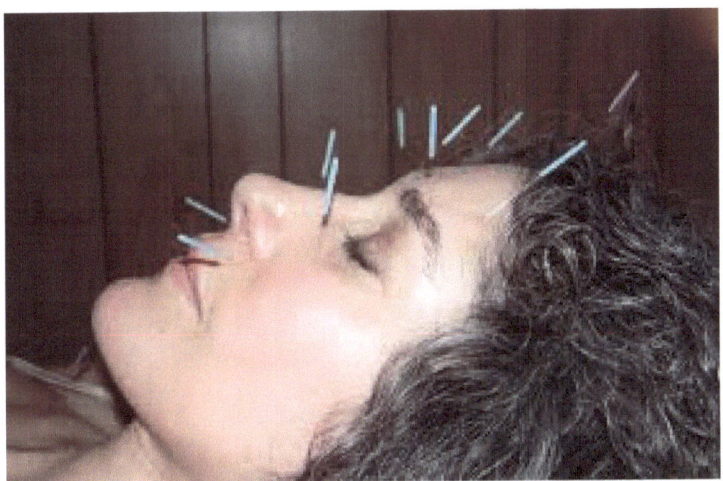

Mixed findings from research. In one study, women who were having moderate to severe hot flushes, who were given acupuncture did benefit. "Individually-tailored acupuncture treatment was associated with significantly greater decrease in the severity, but not the frequency, of hot flushes, when compared to placebo acupuncture," say the researchers from Stanford University in America.

9. Homeopathy

Many homeopathic products can be bought over the counter, but homoeopaths recommend individualised treatment that is matched to the person. Although there have been no well-designed trials for treating menopause symptoms, it has been shown to successfully treat menopause symptoms including flushes and sweats.

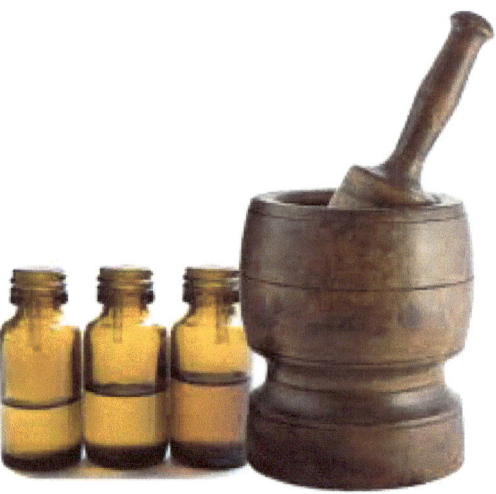

Hypnotic relaxation therapy knocked down hot flashes and other symptoms by up to 80% after 12 weeks, according to a study from Baylor University. The physical relaxation brought on by hypnosis may help settle those brain regions responsible for heat regulation, the study authors hypothesized.

10. Yoga

Make a conscious effort to relax during a hot flush by putting your shoulders down and breathing deeply and slowly. Feeling anxious and stressed often contributes to flushes. In recent years, research has looked at an approach called mindfulness, which includes learning more about the menopause and using relaxation, meditation, yoga and breathing control training. This has shown to be helpful for stress reduction and developing coping strategies.

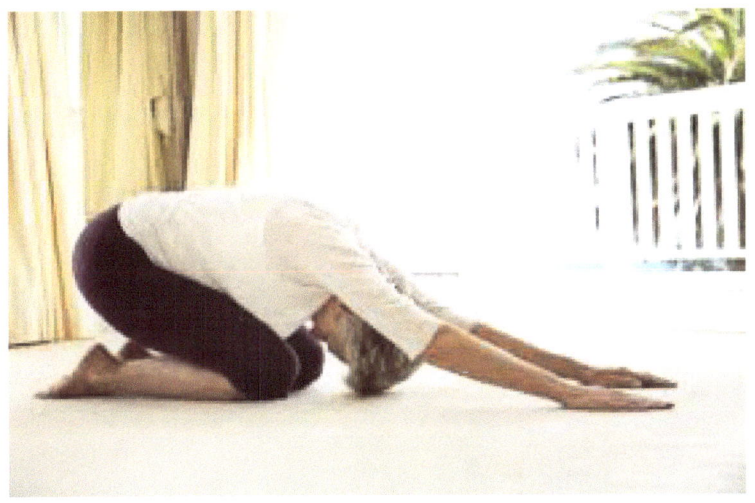

Courses, trainers and books on mindfulness are available. A study at the University of California showed that eight weekly 90-minute sessions led to an average drop in hot flushers each week of 30.8 per cent. The researchers say bigger trials are now needed.

12 Secret Remedies For Night Sweats

1. Black Cohosh

Study results have been mixed about alternative remedies for night sweats, but some women have found relief from symptoms using herbs and supplements such as black cohosh, a native North American plant. To help control hot flashes and night sweats, take 1/2 to 1 mL of black cohosh in tincture form two to four times a day.

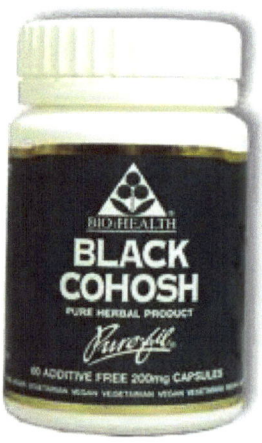

To make it more palatable, add the tincture to half a glass of juice or water. Research has shown that the herb helps control hot flashes by lowering blood levels of luteinizing hormone (LH), which dilates blood vessels and sends heat to the skin. You might get other benefits as well, since some women have found that black cohosh can relieve vaginal dryness, nervousness, and depression. For maximum effectiveness, -take black cohosh for 6 weeks, then take four weeks off before resuming it again. Then repeat the cycle—6 weeks on, 4 weeks off.

2. Vitamin E

Vitamin E is famous for its health benefits to glands and organs, however it may not be generally known that vitamin E is a proven remedy for hot flashes. During the menopause the need for vitamin E soars ten to fifty times over that previously required. Hot flashes and night sweats often disappear when 50 to 500 units of vitamin E are taken daily, but they quickly recur should the vitamin be stopped.

One study supporting vitamin E is from the University of Iran, published in Gynecologic and Obstetric Investigation in 2007. 400 IU of vitamin E in a softgel cap was given to the participants daily for four weeks. A diary was used to measure hot flashes before the study and at the end. The researchers concluded that vitamin E is effective and is a recommended treatment for hot flashes.

3. Flaxseed

Another natural remedy has been making headlines lately. Mayo Clinic breast health specialist Sandhya Pruthi, M.D., conducted a study on flaxseed for hot flashes. The 29 participants in Mayo's clinical trial were women with hot flashes who did not want to take estrogen because of increased risk of breast cancer.

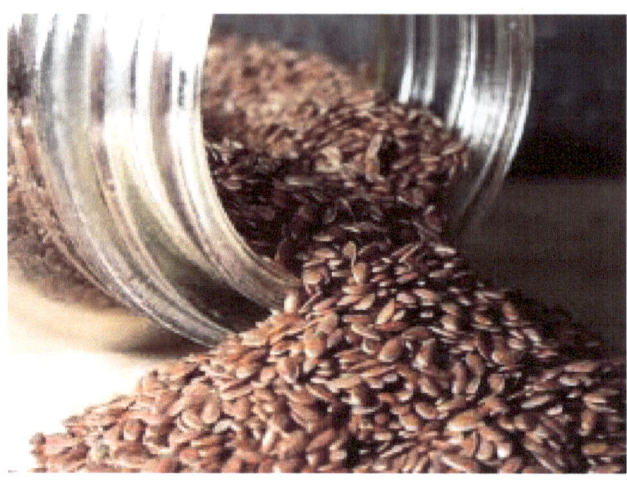

The study gave them six weeks of flaxseed therapy, consisting of 40 grams of crushed flaxseed eaten daily. The result was that the frequency of hot flashes decreased fifty percent.   Participants also reported improvements in mood, joint or muscle pain, chills, and sweating. This was a significant improvement in their health and quality of life. Dr. Pruthi said: "We hope to find more effective nonhormonal options to assist women, and flaxseed looks promising."

4. Pycnogenol

Pycnogenol is a natural plant extract from the bark of the maritime pine tree which grows exclusively along the coast of southwest France. In a study from Taiwan, 100 pre-menopausal women aged 45-55 years, were given 100-mg capsules of Pycnogenol or placebo twice daily (at breakfast and dinner) for 6 months in a double-blind manner.

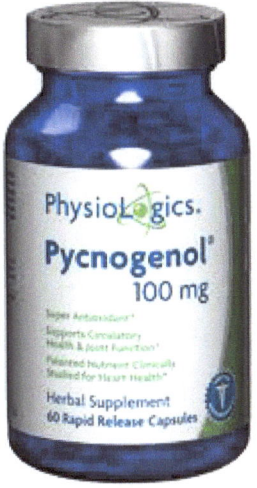

All menopause symptoms evaluated (including depression, hot flashes, night sweats, memory, attractiveness, anxiety, sexual symptoms, and sleep) improved significantly with Pycnogenol treatment, as early as one month after initiation of treatment. The researchers said, "Supplementation with Pycnogenol clearly reduced the frequency as well as the severity of pre-menopausal symptoms."

5. Minerals

Regarding mineral deficiency at the time of menopause, the amount of calcium in a woman's blood parallels the activity of the ovaries. During the menopause, the lack of ovarian hormones (estrogen and progesterone) can cause severe calcium deficiency symptoms to occur, including irritability, hot flashes, night sweats, leg cramps, and insomnia. These problems can be easily overcome if the intakes of calcium, magnesium, and vitamin D are all generously increased and are well absorbed.

One insomnia remedy becoming popular among menopausal women is Sleep Minerals II from Nutrition Breakthroughs. This natural sleep aid contains highly absorbable forms of calcium, magnesium, vitamin D and zinc. The ingredients are formulated with carrier oils such as rice bran oil, an oil that has been shown in studies to lower cholesterol levels, remedy menopause symptoms such as hot flashes and strengthen the immune system.

6. Soy

Besides the obvious choice of eating more fruits and vegetables, eat more soy and fatty acids. Pack in the edamame, tofu and salmon, because they supply the micronutrients you need for hormonal balance. Eat 200 to 250g of tofu every day. Tofu is high in phytoestrogens—compounds with mild estrogen-like qualities that have been found to ease menopausal symptoms. Certain kinds of phytoestrogens, called isoflavones, found in soy products can help ease hot flashes and vaginal dryness. The recommended amount is 60 mg a day of isoflavones, which is what you'll get by eating 200 to 250 g of tofu.

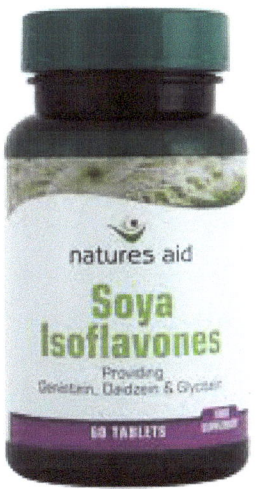

One 50-mg supplement of isoflavones, taken daily, can meet most of your needs when you can't eat a lot of tofu. Look for brands that contain genistein and daidzein.

7. Sage

This is one of the most popular natural remedy recommended for hot flashes, night sweats and insomnia. Studies show us that sage is able to reduce the intensity and frequency of night time sweats by over 50%. A cup of sage tea before bed can make miracles happen. To tame night sweats, take 3 to 15 drops sage tincture three times a day in a half-cup water or tea. The genus name of this herb, Salvia, comes from the Latin salvere (to heal), and the extract of salvia leaves has been used to treat more than 60 different health complaints. The herb has astringent qualities that can help quell profuse sweating.

8. Berries

The berries of the chaste tree have been used by women for some 2,000 years. They help restore progesterone levels, which decrease significantly during menopause.

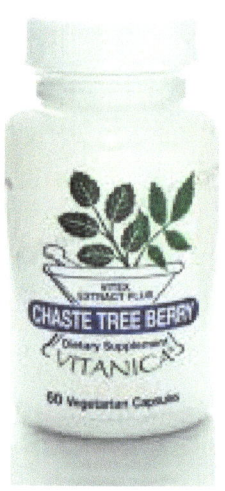

Chaste tree may be particularly useful for combating very heavy bleeding, which some women experience during perimenopause. It may also help with other symptoms, including hot flashes and depression. Take 1 to 2 teaspoons of a standardized extract

9. Teas And Tinctures

Red Clover Tea is a favourite soothing drink during the menopause years and has been used as a tonic for the female reproductive organs. Motherwort tincture has been traditionally used by the Japanese, who claim that it is their secret herb of longevity. Motherwort may help to give support to women experiencing the more intense or volcanic hot flushes. Fenugreek tea is also used as a natural support during menopause and may help to lower the number of flushes during this time. It has been known to make sweat smell of maple syrup!

10. Licorice

Licorice root gives comfort to those affected by insomnia. This herb is rich in glycyrrhizin, a substance that is used for many years in female hormonal disorders. Licorice contains similar estrogen properties that have the power to relieve the symptoms of perimenopause and menopause.

11. Macafem Route

This is a miraculous herb that grows high in the Peruvian mountains. Unlike other plants, macafem feeds the female glands and determines them to produce their own estrogen hormone.

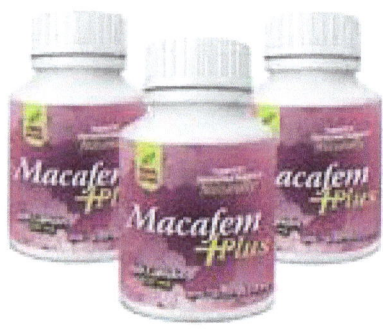

Can you think of a more natural remedy than this? Macafem root eliminates the stress and fights fatigue, headaches and night sweats.

12. Dong Quai

Dong Quai is a root plant that has been used in China and other parts of Asia for thousands of years. It is related to carrots, celery and parsley. It works by balancing hormonal levels of estrogen and progesterone. It also stabilizes your blood vessels, which tones down the sweating.

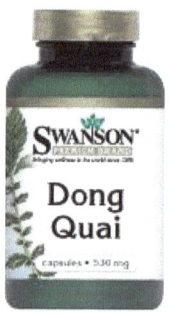

The 10 Most Effective Drugs And Surgical Treatments For Excessive Sweating

1. Hormone Replacement Therapy

Hormone replacement therapy (HRT) is almost always helpful. It works by replacing oestrogen to the levels present pre-menopausally. The problem is that doctors and patients alike are overwhelmed with information about the risks and benefits. In 1991 The National Institute of Health launched the Women's Health Initiative (WHI), the largest clinical trial ever undertaken in the United States. The WHI was designed to provide answers concerning possible benefits and risks associated with use HRT. The findings were published The Journal of the American Medical Association, and to this date have not been disputed.

The big anxiety is breast cancer: does HRT increase the risk? In women aged 50 to 64, the risk of the disease is 32 in every 1,000 women. In those using HRT, there is a slightly higher risk - between 34 and 38 in every 1,000, depending on which study you look at.

The next health hazard is heart disease and stroke, which has been heavily covered in the Press recently. It used to be thought that HRT offered protection against these; but more recent studies not only failed to confirm this, but showed that after an average of five years on HRT, there was a slight increase in heart disease. But again: the numbers are very small - an extra seven cases per 10,000 taking HRT for a year.

Third: Endometrial cancer, or malignant change in the lining of the womb. The increased risk is about three cases in every 1,000 women over five years' observation. Giving women combined HRT (oestrogen plus progestogen) is protective, reducing the incidence to two cases per 1,000 women; but giving oestrogen alone increases the risk to five cases per 1,000, which is why we give HRT as a combination in women who have not had a hysterectomy.

Fourth: Blood clots in veins. There is an increased risk by a factor of two or three when HRT is taken orally, as opposed to being given by skin patches. This is because oral hormones enter the body via the intestine and go straight to the liver, where blood-clotting factors are made. A conflict at that point somehow leads to a change in the blood clotting functions. On a positive note, HRT has beneficial effects on bone strength. Women need oestrogen for good bone health: as the hormone levels decline, the skeleton can weaken. Oestrogen supplementation, therefore, can dramatically reduce the chances of fractures of the hip and spine.

So what's the advice? HRT is not a panacea for all of the ills of middle age, but is worth using to reduce troublesome symptoms such as hot flushes. It should be prescribed in the lowest effective dose, which your doctor will judge. You would see benefits within six weeks and, if not, the dose should be increased.

Generally you'd take HRT for around five years, as by this time the symptoms would have passed, but you should have an annual rethink with your doctor, looking each time at the pros and cons.

If you find that HRT is strictly contra-indicated (for example, you have a history of a deep vein thrombosis), then there is one non-hormonal treatment for hot flushes: the antidepressant drug venalfaxine. This seems to be remarkably effective - though it has none of the other advantages of HRT. It works on the nerve cell communications in the same part of the brain affected by the hot flushes. Make sure you mention your discomfort and concerns to your doctor, who should have all the information about your health history to help you make a balanced judgment.

2. Antidepressants

Low doses of some antidepressants may reduce hot flushes, according to research at the US Mayo Clinic. Selective serotonin re-uptake inhibitors - SSRIs - are among those that have positive effects. Many doctors now consider these anti-depressants the treatment of choice if you have troublesome hot flashes and can't - or choose not to - take hormone therapy. But they aren't as effective as hormone therapy for severe hot flashes and may cause unwanted side effects, such as nausea, dizziness, weight gain or sexual dysfunction.

3. Gabapentin

Gabapentin, an anti-convulsant used for treating seizures and pain associated with shingles, has been shown to reduce symptoms, according to a Wayne State University School of Medicine report, but it is not known how. A study involving 59 women found a reduction of hot flush frequency of 45 per cent compared to 29 per cent for placebo treatment.

4. Clonidine

A pill or patch used to treat high blood pressure, may provide some relief, although there may be side effects including dizziness, drowsiness and dry mouth. According to a Wayne State University School of Medicine study, two small trials found that the pill reduced hot flush frequency by 46 per cent and the patch by 80 per cent.

5. Megestrol Acetate (Megace)

This medication is a type of progesterone, a female hormone. It can be effective in relieving hot flashes, but can only be taken over the short term (for several months). Serious effects can occur if the medication is abruptly discontinued, and megestrol is not usually recommended as a first-line drug to treat hot flashes. Megestrol use can also lead to weight gain.

Studies of another form of progesterone, medroxyprogesterone acetate (Depo-Provera), which is administered by injection, have also shown that this medication can be useful in treating hot flashes. This drug can be used long-term but may have side effects that include weight gain and bone loss.

6. Botox

Many people have found relief from their excessive sweating by receiving Botox injections. This treatment basically shuts down the sweat glands, and has more than a 90% success rate.

7. Sweat Gland Surgery

Sweat gland surgery has been the traditional approach for hyperhidrosis. It consists of removing all or part of the sweat gland. The surgeon may even perform liposuction in the area to cause less disruption to the skin, smaller scars and minimal hairs loss.

8. Endoscopic Thoracic Sympathectomy

Endoscopic Thoracic Sympathectomy is a minimal-invasive endoscopic technique. The operation consists in making a tiny incision in the armpit, and the surgeon identifies and severe the sympathetic nerve-nodes that cause the excessive sweating. This procedure cures nearly 100% of patients, and it only leaves a tiny scar.

9. Lumbar Sympathectomy

When you have excessive sweating in one specific area, especially your palms, lumbar sympathectomy may be an option. It's performed on your back, and it takes about an hour to perform. The success rate for this surgery is about 90%.

10. Local Anesthetics

Sometimes local anesthetics are applied topically as a treatment for excessive sweating. They can block the nerve conduction and reduce sweating, but they are not highly effective. Also, you can develop hypersensitivity as you continue to use them.